Mental Wellness Strategies.

Transform Your Life: Practical Strategies for Optimal Mental Wellness.

By

Rhonda J. Williams

TABLE OF CONTENT

Introduction

Navigating the Path to Optimal Mental Wellness

Welcome to a transformative odyssey — "Mental Wellness Strategies: Empower Your Mind, Transform Your Life." In the tapestry of our fast-paced lives, this book unfolds as a guide, a companion, and an invitation to embark on a journey toward lasting well-being

As we stand at the intersection of the everyday and the extraordinary, this book beckons you to explore the depths of your mental landscape. The title is not just a promise; it's a roadmap to empower your mind and transform your life. In the pages that follow, we navigate the intricacies of understanding mental wellness, tapping into your inner power, and crafting a personalized plan that transcends theory to become your lived reality.

This isn't just another self-help book; it's a collection of insights, strategies, and real-life stories carefully woven to resonate with the complexities of your journey. Each chapter is a stepping stone, guiding you toward a more resilient, empowered, and balanced version of yourself.

So, open these pages with curiosity and anticipation. Let this be more than a read; let it be an immersive experience, a dialogue between the words on the page and the aspirations within you. Welcome to a journey where understanding meets action, where challenges transform into opportunities, and where the pursuit of optimal mental wellness becomes a lifelong adventure. The voyage begins now.

Chapter 1

Welcome to Your Mental Wellness Journey

Welcome, dear reader, to a transformative voyage — your Mental Wellness Journey. In these pages, we embark together on a profound exploration of the intricate tapestry that is your mental well-being. This book is not just a guide; it's an invitation to discover the power within you and to transform the way you navigate the complexities of modern life.

Acknowledging the Struggles of Modern Living

In a world marked by constant change and ever-increasing demands, acknowledging the struggles is the first step towards growth. This chapter compassionately recognizes the challenges that accompany the fast-paced nature of our contemporary existence. From the pressures of career and relationships to the digital noise that fills our daily lives, we stand together at the threshold of understanding and overcoming these challenges.

This isn't just a book; it's a conversation about embracing the full spectrum of your experiences. By acknowledging these struggles, we lay the groundwork for a journey that goes beyond mere survival. It's about thriving amidst the chaos, finding balance in the midst of upheaval, and reclaiming a sense of peace that is rightfully yours.

So, as we turn the pages together, let this be more than a read — let it be an immersive experience, a guide, and a companion on your path to mental wellness. Welcome to a journey where self-discovery meets practical wisdom, where acknowledgment is the first step towards transformation.

Chapter 2

Understanding the Essence of Mental Wellness

Welcome to the heart of our exploration — Chapter 2, where we delve into the very essence of Mental Wellness. Here, we embark on a thoughtful journey to unravel the intricacies that define a healthy state of mind.

Defining Mental Wellness and Its Components

At its core, mental wellness is more than the absence of illness; it's a holistic state encompassing emotional, psychological, and social well-being. In this chapter, we dissect this definition, exploring the multifaceted components that contribute to a truly balanced mental state. From emotional intelligence to cognitive resilience, we'll navigate the various dimensions that form the foundation of your well-being.

Recognizing the Interconnectedness of Mind and Body

A crucial aspect often overlooked is the symbiotic relationship between the mind and body. As we unravel the threads of mental wellness, we'll explore how physical health, emotional balance, and cognitive harmony are intertwined. Understanding this interconnectedness is pivotal, for it lays the groundwork for practical strategies that bridge the gap between mental and physical well-being.

So, join me in Chapter 2 as we unravel the essence of mental wellness — a journey that goes beyond definitions, inviting you to discover the profound and interconnected nature of your own mind. It's not just about understanding; it's about laying the groundwork for a transformative experience that will resonate through the entirety of your Mental Wellness Journey.

Chapter 3:

Unleashing Your Inner Power

Welcome to Chapter 3, where the pages come alive with the promise of discovery and empowerment. Here, we embark on a journey of self-realization, tapping into the reservoirs of strength that reside within you. Tapping into Your Personal Potential In the tapestry of your being, there exists untapped potential waiting to be unleashed. This chapter serves as a guide to unearth and harness that inner power. Together, we'll explore exercises and reflections designed to reveal the unique strengths that make you who you are. Through self-discovery, you'll find the keys to unlocking a reservoir of capabilities you may not have fully recognized.

Identifying and Overcoming Limiting Beliefs Often, our most formidable barriers are the beliefs we hold about ourselves. In this section, we confront these limiting beliefs head-on. Through practical strategies and insightful exercises, you'll learn to identify and challenge thoughts that hinder your progress. By doing so, you open the door to a transformative process where self-imposed limitations give way to a newfound sense of personal agency.

So, let's dive into Chapter 3 — an exploration of self-discovery and empowerment. As we navigate the terrain of your inner power, remember, this journey is not just about reading words; it's about internalizing the wisdom within them. Get

ready to unleash the extraordinary potential
that resides within you.

Chapter 4:

Daily Practices for Optimal Well-Being

Welcome to Chapter 4, a compass guiding you towards the integration of practical strategies into your daily life for sustained well-being.

Mindful Living: Incorporating Daily Mindfulness

In the hustle of our daily lives, the practice of mindfulness becomes a transformative anchor. This chapter illuminates the art of mindful living, offering practical insights on seamlessly integrating mindfulness into your routine. Through simple yet powerful exercises, you'll learn to cultivate a present-focused mindset, fostering a sense of clarity and peace amid life's chaos.

Nurturing Healthy Habits for a Balanced Life

The fabric of your well-being is woven with the threads of daily habits. This section explores the science of habit formation and guides you in nurturing habits that contribute to a balanced and fulfilling life. From cultivating a healthy sleep routine to incorporating movement into your day, these habits are the building blocks of sustained well-being.

As we delve into Chapter 4, envision it as a toolkit for daily empowerment. It's not just about reading; it's about actively participating in the transformation of your daily life. Get ready to embrace mindful living and cultivate habits that will lay the

foundation for your journey towards
optimal well-being.

Chapter 5

Cultivating a Transformative Mindset

Welcome to Chapter 5, a transformative juncture in your Mental Wellness Journey.Here, we embark on the dynamic exploration of cultivating a mindset that not only adapts but propels you toward positive transformation.

Embracing a Positive Mindset
In the landscape of mental wellness, your mindset is the compass that guides your journey. This chapter unfolds the art of embracing a positive mindset, illuminating the profound impact it can have on your overall well-being. Through insightful discussions and practical exercises, you'll learn to navigate challenges with optimism,

fostering a mindset that sees opportunities in every obstacle.

Embracing Change as a Catalyst for Personal Growth

Change is the only constant, and in this section, we redefine it as a catalyst for personal growth. Together, we'll explore how embracing change can become a powerful force in your life. By shifting your perspective on change, you'll not only weather life's inevitable storms but also harness their energy for personal evolution. This chapter lays the groundwork for a mindset that thrives on adaptability and resilience.

So, join me in Chapter 5 — a chapter that transcends mere positivity and delves into the art of cultivating a transformative mindset. It's a journey of redefining challenges, embracing change, and forging a mental landscape that propels you toward the life you aspire to lead. Get ready to shift your mindset and unlock the door to profound personal growth.

Chapter 6

Breaking Through Mental Roadblocks

Step into Chapter 6, a guide that empowers you to navigate and conquer the mental roadblocks that stand between you and your optimal well-being.

Strategies for Dealing with Stress and Anxiety

In the ever-evolving tapestry of life, stress and anxiety often weave their threads. This chapter serves as a compass, offering practical strategies to not only cope with but transcend these challenges. Through mindfulness techniques, stress management tools, and actionable insights, you'll gain the resilience to face adversity with a calm and centered mind.

Building Resilience in the Face of
Challenges

eveloping adaptive strategies, you'll emerge
from difficulties with newfound strength
and a deeper understanding of your own
resilience.

As you embark on Chapter 6, envision it as a
guide through the labyrinth of mental
challenges. It's not just about overcoming
obstacles; it's about emerging stronger on
the other side. Get ready to break through
mental roadblocks, paving the way for a
more resilient and empowered version of
yourself.

Chapter 7

Lifestyle Choices and Mental Wellness

Step into Chapter 7, a pivotal exploration into the profound impact that lifestyle choices wield on your mental wellness.
The Impact of Nutrition and Exercise
The food you eat and the movement you engage in are not just elements of your daily routine; they are fundamental pillars of mental well-being. This chapter delves into the intricate connection between nutrition, exercise, and your mental state. Through practical advice and evidence-based insights, you'll gain a holistic understanding of how nourishing your body positively influences your mind.

Creating a Supportive Environment

Your surroundings play a significant role in shaping your mental landscape. This section guides you in crafting a supportive environment conducive to mental well-being. From decluttering physical spaces to

fostering positive relationships, we explore the art of creating a life-enhancing backdrop that nurtures your mental health.

As you immerse yourself in Chapter 7, envision it as a roadmap to a lifestyle that harmonizes with your mental well-being goals. It's not just about making choices; it's about creating an environment that uplifts and sustains your mental health. Get ready to align your lifestyle with your aspirations for optimal mental wellness.

Chapter 8

The Role of Relationships in Mental Wellness

Step into Chapter 8, a compelling exploration into the intricate dance between relationships and your mental well-being. Building and Nurturing Meaningful Connections
Relationships form the fabric of our lives, influencing our emotions, thoughts, and overall mental state. This chapter delves into the art of building and nurturing meaningful connections. Through practical insights and heartfelt discussions, you'll discover how genuine connections can be a source of strength, providing support and

companionship on your journey to optimal mental wellness.

Navigating Relationship Challenges for Mental Well-Being

Challenges within relationships are inevitable, but how we navigate them can profoundly impact our mental health. This section offers guidance on navigating relationship challenges with resilience and empathy. By fostering effective communication and understanding, you'll not only overcome obstacles but also cultivate relationships that contribute positively to your mental well-being. Consider Chapter 8 to be a compass guiding you across the perilous landscape of human interactions. It's not only about the people in your life; it's about cultivating relationships that raise and nourish your mental health. Prepare to delve into the important significance that connections have in constructing your mental environment.

Chapter 9

Actual Success Stories

Welcome to Chapter 9, a thrilling journey into the remarkable stories of people who have overcome mental health challenges. Inspiring Stories of Overcoming Mental Health Difficulties
to explore the profound role relationships play in shaping your mental landscape. Inspiring Tales of Overcoming Mental Health Struggles
In the tapestry of personal growth, real-life stories are the threads that weave inspiration and hope. This chapter brings you authentic and uplifting tales of individuals who have navigated and transcended mental health challenges.

Through their experiences, you'll find relatable examples of resilience, courage, and the transformative power of implementing the strategies discussed throughout this book.

Highlighting the Transformational Power of the Strategies

Each success story serves as a testament to the effectiveness of the strategies explored in earlier chapters. By showcasing real people who have applied these principles in their lives, this section aims to reinforce the belief that positive change is not only possible but achievable. These stories illuminate the transformative power of embracing a mental wellness journey.

As you immerse yourself in Chapter 9, envision it as a collection of beacons lighting the way through the challenges of mental health. It's not just about the stories; it's about discovering that your journey is shared by many. Get ready to be inspired and motivated by real-life success stories that resonate with the authenticity of human experience.

Chapter 10

Crafting Your Personal Mental Wellness Plan

Welcome to Chapter 10, a transformative guide where theory meets action, and you embark on the creation of a personalized roadmap to lasting mental well-being. Developing a Tailored Plan for Lasting Results

In this chapter, we transition from insights to implementation, guiding you in crafting a personalized mental wellness plan. Drawing on the principles and strategies explored throughout the book, you'll engage in practical exercises to identify your unique goals and aspirations. This section is designed to empower you to take ownership

of your mental well-being, ensuring the
sustainability of positive changes in your
life.

Empowering Readers to Take Concrete
Actions

Knowledge alone is not enough; it's the
actions we take that shape our reality. This
section provides actionable steps and
frameworks to translate the insights gained
into tangible changes. By the end of Chapter
10, you'll have a clear and actionable mental
wellness plan, empowering you to integrate
these strategies seamlessly into your daily
life.

As you delve into Chapter 10, see it as the
culmination of your journey — the moment
you become the architect of your mental
well-being. It's not just about
understanding; it's about doing. Get ready

to craft a plan that aligns with your goals, values, and vision for a life marked by sustained mental wellness.

Chapter 11

Conclusion

Your Continued JourneyIn the concluding chapter, we stand at the crossroads of reflection and anticipation — Chapter 11, your bridge between the journey so far and the path that stretches ahead.

Recapitulation and Reinforcement of Key Concepts

As we look back on the chapters that have unfolded, this section serves as a compass, guiding you through a recapitulation of key concepts. It's an opportunity to revisit the insights and strategies that have shaped your understanding of mental wellness. Through this review, we reinforce the foundation upon which your continued journey is built.

Encouragement for the Journey Ahead

Beyond the pages of this book lies the ongoing adventure of your personal growth. This chapter is not an endpoint but a launching pad for your continued journey. With words of encouragement and support, you're invited to embrace the path ahead, equipped with newfound wisdom and a personalized mental wellness plan. Your journey doesn't conclude here; it extends into the limitless possibilities that await.

As you conclude this book, envision Chapter 11 as a stepping stone to your ongoing evolution. It's not just about finishing a chapter; it's about embarking on the next phase of your transformative journey. Get ready to carry the lessons, insights, and empowerment garnered here into the chapters of your life yet to be written. Your continued journey to optimal mental wellness begins.

Thank you as you do so.

9 798887 493953